Medicinal Herbs

20 Herbs to Grow in Your Kitchen All Year Round!

Table of Contents

Introduction

I would like to thank and congratulate you for downloading *"Medicinal Herbs: Effective Medicinal Herbs You Can Grow in Your Own Kitchen Garden!"* This is a great step you are taking towards living a more natural and healthy lifestyle.

Many people are turning to more natural options in the food and medicinal choices they are making. People are beginning to realize just how much more beneficial the all-natural choices are in our lives. These choices will effect our overall health and well-being so we want to make sure that we are making the right healthy choices in life.

A great way for you to help ensure that you have natural medicinal herbs for your use is to grow them yourself. This will release you from depending on other sources to supply you with your medicinal herbs and it is also going to save you a lot of money compared to buying them from others.

This guide is very easy to follow I can assure you that you will be growing your amazing medicinal herbs in no time at all! The great thing is that you do not have to have a large outside garden, you can even grow your own medicinal herbs in pots inside your home.

Even if you are living in an apartment you can still make a little space by a window perhaps in your kitchen to grow your favorite medicinal herbs.

In this book we are going to scratch the surface of the many uses of some of the most commonly used herbs and how to grow them. The information in this book will offer you knowledge on the world of medicinal plants. If you are someone that is planning to live off the grid then having your own medicinal garden will certainly be a good addition to this lifestyle.

Chapter 1. Why Grow Medicinal Herbs?

There is a vast array of reasons why people would consider growing medicinal herbs. It does not matter where you live whether you live in the country, city or suburbs the benefits of herbal medicines will be the same.

You will be able to solve a whole assorted range of small medical nuisances, as well as producing your own healing cosmetic products. You can become more self-sufficient by growing your own medicinal herbs and less dependant on pharmacy drugs. Using the homegrown natural products will draw you closer to nature. Gaining knowledge about the common plants and herbs that can help to keep you healthy will be invaluable to you.

You can look at the medicinal herbs covered in this book as supplements to traditional pharmaceutical medicines. However, you should always consult with your physician when you are dealing with serious medical conditions or a long-term medical issue. For the simple health issues such as headaches, muscle pain or a simple flu, it can be very helpful to give natural herbal remedies a try.

Other common uses for medicinal herbs as being great to use for basic cosmetic products is another reason people are drawn to growing medicinal plants. Using herbal plants to make natural herbal cosmetics is a healthy alternative to the products that are offered at stores that are often full of ingredients that are synthetic.

The medicinal herbs that we will cover in this book are easy to grow and will not require much effort to produce them. You will find it easy to follow the steps in this book towards you growing your own little medicinal herbal garden. You do not need to own a big farm in order to grow your medicinal herb garden, a few pots will do the trick!

If you are an aspiring herbalist looking to grow medicinal herbs as a long-term natural alternative to expensive medicinal products then you will enjoy following the tips and suggestions in this book. They will help get you started on the road to becoming a well-seasoned herbalist in no time!

You might want to produce your own soaps and shampoos or use natural alternatives to expensive painkillers, and inflammatory pills for example. Following the steps within this books pages you will be able to understand the uses and caretaking processes for the medicinal plants that you want to grow more fully.

Growing your own medicinal garden will give you the opportunity to use the natural healing powers of these medicinal herbs to improve your life. Over thousands of years the healing powers of these plants has strengthened. Taking a look into the history of medicinal herbs applications will also help you to better understand you are drawn to learn about and grow medicinal herbs.

Chapter 2. A Brief Glimpse Into the History of Medicinal Herbs

When we look back through time we can see that there has been a natural evolution between humans and medicinal plants that have been useful to them. The knowledge of uses of herbal plants have been passed down from generation to generation, until recently when more people began to resort more to synthetic pharmaceutical solutions as opposed to natural medicinal benefits of herbal plants.

Due to the rise in the amounts of modern day medical facilities our collective knowledge of herbalism is unfortunately on the decline. Until recently that is with the sprouting of those seeking to take a more sustainable option and resort back to traditional herbal methods.

Human Medicinal Roots

Looking back through the human timeline there is basically not a point in time when we were not applying some type of natural solution to our health issues. When we humans were hunter-gatherers we sought after natural products, especially medicinal herbal plants, using them to treat many different health problems.

As time passed our knowledge of the most useful and common herbs became institutionalized into our culture. The knowledge has continued to be passed down through the generations. We can look back in history as far back as the Paleolithic era as being the time of earliest evidence of medicinal plant usage in human history. That is a point in time going back about 60,000 years ago. Our long history with medicinal herbs show how deep-rooted our connection is to medicinal plants.

The first written evidence dates back 5000 years it is Mesoptamian of using medicinal herbs to treat our ailments. In the bible you will find that over a hundred different types of herbs are mentioned in it. This is proof of how important medicinal herbs were in cultures several millennia ago.

Books and texts became more common in the Middle Ages with detailed descriptions along with biologically accurate drawings of medicinal plants. Many of the books that had the knowledge of medicinal herbs was kept in monasteries. This shows a clear historical connection between religion and herbalism knowledge. Embedding herbalism into religious beliefs was a way of keeping the knowledge alive.

Decline Begins

During the period of history when the black plague took a significant death toll in medieval societies was when the real turnaround time began regarding the popularity of herbal solutions. People during this time began to realize that the healing properties of medicinal plants were not going to stop them from getting this horrible disease. This began the decline of overall trust in medicinal herbs as a healing method.

During this time period is when other strange practices were happening such as bloodletting were popular. With the introduction of modern medical solutions herbal solutions soon took a back seat, and were viewed as an alternative solution to modern medicine solutions.

Herbalism in Modern Times

The modern-day pharmaceutical industry has pretty much got the strong-hold as the main supplier of medical solutions to the world. The World Health Organization has estimated that over 80% of people are using some form of herbal medicine in their daily lives.

People are using plant-based medicines with and without prescriptions. It is showing that the treatments using herbal products is on the rise. These herbal products are being viewed as a viable alternative that will have less negative side effects and they have low production costs.

Chapter 3. Most Common Medicinal Herb—Lavender

Lavender is one of the most common medicinal herbs that can be found around the world. Lavender is also called *Lavandula* with its most common species *Lavandula angusttifolia,* this is the Latin name for the plant that belongs to the mint family that is called *Lamiaceae.* Many people love to use lavender in culinary dishes. The extraction of the essential oils of lavender plants is used for medicinal purposes, basically offering an alternative natural remedy to some common health problems.

Introduction to Lavender

You can easily spot lavender with its lovely bright purple flower and long thin green stem. Nectar loving creatures love the lavender nectar. Lavender has a wide assortment of practical uses but it is also great addition to your garden as it is visually appealing. There is many different subspecies of lavender found in the *Lamiaceae* family.

The common differences are the shapes of their leaves, these have hairs on them which collect the essential oils. The species that are the most cultivated have these hairs on them, there is other subspecies that do not have these hairs. The shape and color of the flower can differ slightly. You can find it in variations of violet, purple, blackish, blue and yellow, all with their own slight differences in the shape of their flowers. The most common species that is cultivated is the English lavender. Shown here in this picture.

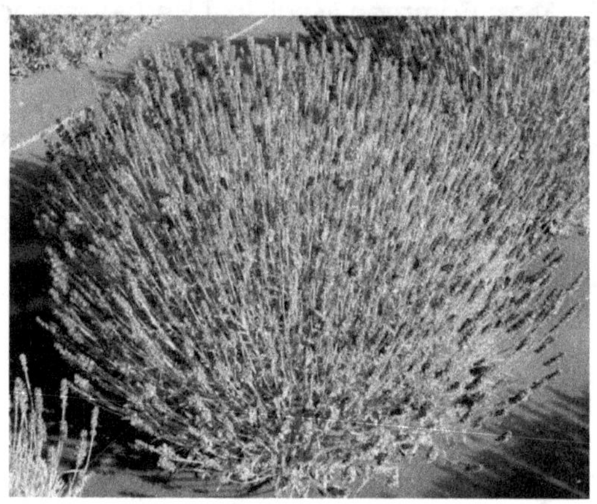

English Lavender

How to Grow

When it comes to growing lavender it is not too complicated. You can buy these plants in most gardening stores as semi-grown, full-grown or seeds. Lavender plants have very few requirements, so as a beginner you should have no problems growing lavender. I have outlined an easy 5-step process for you to follow.

Step 1: Soil Preparation

You want to find the right location for your lavender plants. Look for an area that is well-lit—has plenty of natural sunlight. If you are growing it in a pot make sure the pot you choose as proper drainage possibilities. Lavender roots should not get over-hydrated as they are highly sensitive to excess water in their system.

You need to check the pH-level of your soil. You should use a soil with a pH-level around 7. This you can easily check with the pH-strips you can get at garden shops. If you find that the soil is good then dig a small hole in the middle, enough to fit the roots into and fit the plant into it.

Using two handfuls of round stone and half a cup of a mixture of lime and manure or similar fertilizer. Add the stones to bottom of pot to aide with water drainage. The lime and manure mix will offer growth support also making sure that the soil is alkalized correctly. Add these mixtures to the bottom of the hole you made to put lavender in. Cover mix up with a layer of regular soil, you do not want the roots to come in contact with mixes.

Step 2: Pot Preparation

First you should water the lavender in the nursery pot that you purchased it in. Once it has been watered prune the plant. Lightly prune your lavender plant along the sides. This will help stimulate the internal air circulation and it is a vital step in stimulating growth. It will also help to prevent wooding within the center of the plant. Lavender has a tendency to wooden up at the base of plant pruning will help to avoid this issue. Remove from nursery pot and remove the soil from roots. Introducing the plant to a new soil environment will help stimulate growth and adaptation process. This is a crucial step in regards to long-term growth success of your lavender.

Step 3: Planting your lavender

Place your lavender roots into the prepared hole in the soil. Make sure that the roots do not come in contact with stone and fertilizer mix. Fill layer of normal soil between this mix and the lavender roots. Make sure that you leave a space between lavender plants of about 35 inches so that they will have optimal growth and air circulation.

Step 4: Lavender Maintenance

You may want to try using a fish or seaweed extract mixture to add onto the soil surrounding your lavender plant during the summer or extra summer fertilization. Use the fertilizer mix mentioned earlier in the spring of each year.

 In general lavender is low-maintenance, it does not require much of your help after you have planted it. You do not want to over water your lavender plant as this will kill it quicker than a drought would. The most common way lavender plants die is from people over watering them. Lavender is very sensitive to excess hydration.

Step 5: Harvesting

The best time to harvest your lavender is when the bottom flowers are starting to open up. This will assure that the plant is fresh and that the accumulated essential oils are ready to harvest to make use of in medicinal remedies. Cut the flowers near the stems base. You may choose to dry them in bundles tied together using a rubber band. Keep bundles indoors in a warm and dark part of the house. Suspend them upside down for about two weeks. Hang them on a nail.

The essential oils can be extracted through the use of steam distillation. You can do this at home using a pan and some heat and water. Check out online different processes in detail.

Health Applications of Lavender

There is over a dozen known health applications that Lavender oil is used in. Some of the common medicinal applications of lavender oil are the following:

Aches and pain:

Having a bath with some lavender oil added into it will help your aching muscles feel so much better after a long hard day at work. The lavender oil will help to relieve your sore muscle tissues.

Fever reduction:

With kids that are suffering from a severe fever you can add a few drops of lavender oil in water at body temperature this will provide an aide that will help reduce the effects of the fever. It will also help the child sleep better at night. Prepare a tepid lavender bath before they go to bed.

Acne and Eczema treatment:

Lavender oil has strong antibacterial properties and can help reduce harmful bacteria on skin and will also moisturize skin.

Soothes Earache:

Lavender is an ideal solution for relieving ear pain. Massage a few drops of lavender oil around the outside of ear. This can also be applied around throat area. The pain sensations throughout the face will be reduced and will help speed up the healing process.

Reduce stress in mind and muscle:

Lavender oil is great at helping to relieve stress. It is often used in tepid water or hot water baths, you can also apply a few drops around the temples, forehead, and neck to reduce headache effects and help trigger a calmness of the mind and head muscles.

Fighting motion sickness:

Apply a mixture of lavender oil, sage and rosemary essential oils to your pulse points to help reduce nausea. Your pulse points are areas of your body where you can easily detect your heart beat such as the inside of your wrists.

Heal cuts and bruises:

You can apply lavender oil to a bruised area or paper cut to remove the burning sensation. The strong antibacterial properties of the oil will help reduce your chances of infection.

Menstrual cramp reduction:

Apply some lavender oil near the areas that are cramping and it will help to reduce the pain.

Fight off insects including scabies: Bugs that are after your blood and like to sting you do not like the smell and taste of lavender oil. Put some drops of lavender oil in a spray bottle with distilled water and spray your body with this solution to keep the pesky bugs away. Lavender oil works great at fighting scabies, these are tiny bugs that borrow into skin. These can become life-threatening if untreated.

Chapter 4. Medicinal Herbs: Thyme & Marigold

Thyme is a herb that has many practical uses. You can make use of the essential oils and the leaves of this plant. The essential oil is mostly used for medicinal purposes, the leaves of the plant are used in culinary dishes. It is also a popular ornamental plant. Humans have been using them way back to ancient civilization when Egyptians used it in their embalming process, and Greeks like to use it in their bathhouses. Romans used it to add flavor to alcoholic beverages and cheeses.

Herbalists go after the working ingredient in it called *thymol,* this composites about 20-50% of the essential oil. If you use or have used mouth wash such as Listerine then there is a good chance that thyme was one of the ingredients. It is a very strong antiseptic herb. It is ideal for many medicinal purposes.

How to grow Thyme

You will find thyme thriving in hot sunny places with soil that is well-drained. It is a fairly sturdy plant and can grow pretty much anywhere that the sun is shining. It will remain green throughout the seasons. Just like lavender does. The best time to plant your thyme is in the Spring. Thyme does not need a lot of watering.

It is recommended that you water them enough during the planting process. Make sure that the soil you plant them in is well-drained. You can use a similar soil mix as what you would use for lavender. Thyme can be grown close together and thrive in the full sun. You may need to give it some slight pruning once a year in the springtime. Prune the plant at points where you can see new growth growing. This process will help stimulate the process of new growth. You can keep trimming the tips off up until the first frost period comes. You do not need to worry about constant watering with your thyme plant.

In cold climate weather you can help stop your thyme plant from freezing by adding a thin layer of gravel or sand onto the soil. Spray the plants lightly with a mix of water and some rosemary essential oil to keep away the spider mites or use a water and soap solution.

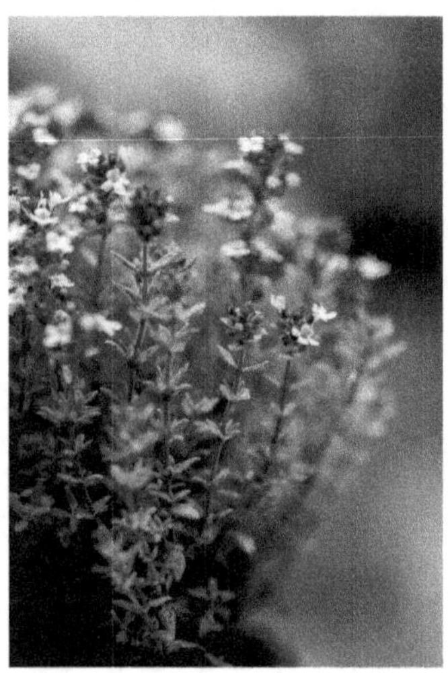

Harvesting thyme

You can harvest your thyme as you need it. You can preserve thyme in numerous ways such as drying them in a bundle or freeze them for example.

Health applications

Thyme is a favorite taste maker used in many culinary dishes, but it also has a range of health benefits. You can usually obtain them through using thyme essential oil. Some of the health benefits of thyme are the following:

Lowers blood pressure:

Within thyme the working components help in reducing the heart rate when having high blood pressure. Other studies have suggested that thyme may also help to reduce or lower cholesterol in the blood. You can use it as a replacement for salt in your food.

Stops coughing and soothes sore throats

Thyme essential oils help to loosen up the lung tissue. Thyme essential oil is used mostly in cough medicines.

Immunity booster:

Thyme is a great source of vitamins A, and C as well as manganese, copper, iron and fibers.

Anti-bacterial and antiviral properties

Thyme essential oil is great at keeping mold away. It has strong disinfecting properties. The strong anti-fungal properties that thyme oil contains will help you to get rid of mold once and for all. It will help keep the viruses and bacteria away.

Enhances mood:

The active substance carvacrol found in thyme is a therapeutic substance that can actively alter neurons in your brain. Studies have shown that this substance can alter mood when it is used in an aromatic substance within your home.

Disinfects and provides refreshing aroma:

Thyme oil has wonderful disinfectant properties. Is used in many cosmetic products.

Marigold

Marigolds will thrive well in moderate or warm climates. They are a sturdy and hardy plant that you can plant after the last frost. Best to plant in morning or cloudy day. They don't mind having about 20% shade but they love the sun. They need to have sunlight.

You may choose to put marigold in your flowerbed or your herbal garden as a herb or even in a pot. Make sure they are about 2 feet apart. Dig to about six inches and break up the soil to ensure oxygen is taken up by the top layer of soil. Follow the five step procedure I mentioned earlier in the book in chapter 3. The hydration process for marigold is pretty similar to that of lavender.

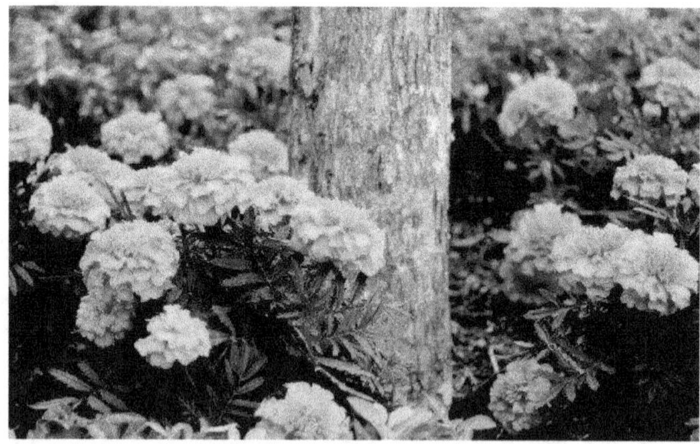

Health applications:

The extracts of the marigold flower serve a multitude of purposes, the essential oils are a great addition to the medicine cabinet in any home. Some of the health-related applications are the following:

Heals cuts and bruises:

The anti-biotic properties found in the marigold flower help heal cuts and bruises. It serves basically as a blood vessel regrowth accelerator. Studies have shown that when a little marigold essential oil is applied to a wound the skin heals much faster.

Fights against warts and skin infections:

The marigold flower is strongly anti-inflammatory, which can help fight warts and other infections. Crush the flower and use the juice to apply to warts or skin infections.

Slows ageing:

The antioxidants that marigold contains helps to prevent free radicals from being created, this in turn slows the ageing process down. Add some marigold extract to your tea.

Helps fight against bladder infections:

Due to the antibiotic and anti-inflammatory properties of the marigold flower these help fight off infections in the bladder and allow the tissue to heal faster.

Eye wash:

There is wonderful healing components called *lutein zeaxanthin & lycopene* are good at helping to prevent eye infections. Use marigold extract as an eyewash.

Detoxifies the body:

The marigold flower stimulates the lymph system in the body and removes toxic agents away from your lymphomas.

Fights bowel disease and cancers:

Drinking marigold tea can help fight against bowel disease and certain cancers.

Chapter 5. Medicinal Herbs—Rosemary, Aloe Vera & Lemon Balm

Rosemary

This is a wonderful plant that offers you anti-bacterial and anti-inflammatory properties. The wonderful aroma of this plant will make your home smell clean and refreshed.

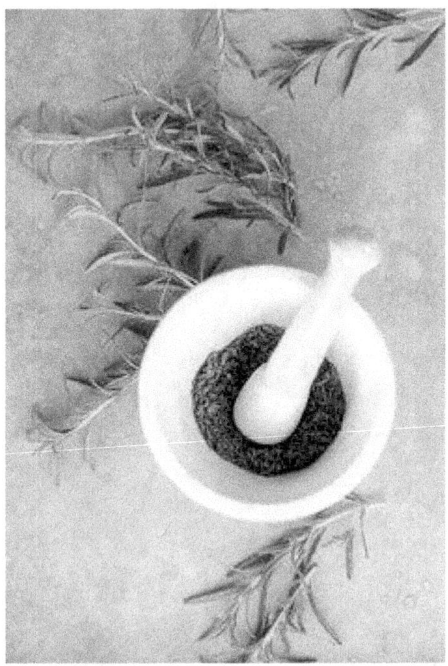

How to grow

The quickest way that you can grow rosemary is to use the cutting of another plant, instead of growing it from seed. Get a little bundle of cuttings and they will grow into a fully grown plant quickly. When planting cuttings put them into a pot that is 2/3 full of coarse soil and sand along with 1/3 of peat moss. Place them deep enough into soil so they do not fall out.

Place pot in spot where there is plenty of sunshine. Water the soil daily and do not keep plant in full blazing sun but in a relatively warm spot. Once the roots have formed, you can place the plant in a bigger pot or in the garden. It is a hardy plant be able to survive most weather types, does really well in hot and dry climates.

It will generally live off rainwater as it prefers dry soil. You can water it infrequently when the soil becomes too dry. Prune plants when they are getting too big. You can harvest the plant all year round. Cut off the tops of the plants only. Keep the sprigs in a dry cool place such as your fridge. For long term storage keep in the freezer. Place harvest in freezer bags and store. Rosemary can be used in culinary dishes as well as a health product.

Health applications

You can use the essential oils from rosemary for a range of different health problems. You should always dilute it when taking it, and is not meant to take orally in concentrated form.

Helps to relieve stress and improve mood:

In the practice of aromatherapy rosemary is often used. It has been scientifically proven that the aromatic benefits can improve overall mood, and relieve stress. It can also help with hormonal problems and help to clear the mind.

Boost memory:

The rosemary herb can help to boost the retention of memory. Scientists have also observed rosemary's active ingredients in stimulating cognitive capacities in elderly people who suffer from dementia or Alzheimer's disease.

Strengthens the immune system:

Rosemary essential oil is great at helping to aid the immune system in fighting off harmful intruders in our bodies. The antioxidant effects of rosemary essential oil will help serve as a second defence.

Antibacterial and Anti-inflammatory:

This wonderful herb helps also in the fighting off diseases due to its anti-bacterial and anti-inflammatory properties.

Aloe Vera

The aloe vera plant is one of the most common plants that is used in many cosmetic products. It also has a nice range of health benefits to it as well. This plant offers an impressive list of helpful substances such as Vitamin A, B1, B2, B6, B12, C, and E, it also contains minerals aluminum, calcium, calcium-oxalate, chloride, chrome, cobalt, phosphorous, potassium, copper, iron, sodium, tin, selenium, manganese, and zinc.

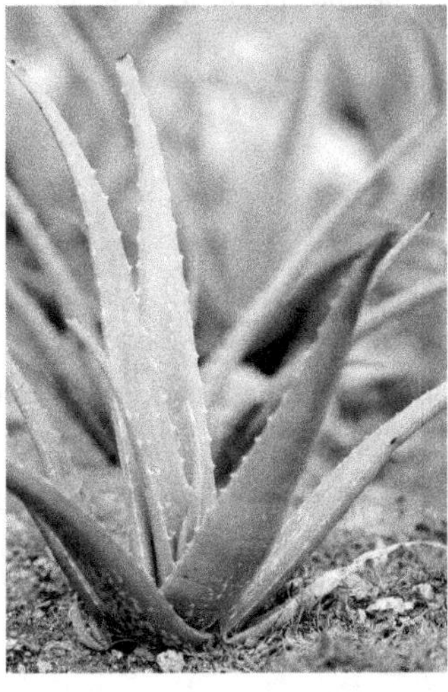

How to grow

This is a great choice for one of your first herb species in plants as it is very easy to grow. You can actually grow a new plant from a single leaf. All you need would be the leaf, a clay pot with some large holes, potting soil and some fertilizer, watering hose, a fragment of broken pottery, a spoon, and a knife.

First you prepare the clay pot. It should have at least one large hole in the bottom. Take the piece of broken pottery and place it over the hole. This will allow the water to flow through and the soil to remain in the pot. Fill the pot with a mix of soil and a fertilizer of your choice.

Place the aloe vera leaf horizontally into the soil. You should still leave the top of leaf exposed. Place pot in sunlight and water it. Fill pot with water and allow to drain. In about four weeks time you will see your leaf sprouting new leaves beginning a new plant.

When the plant is mature then you can take the knife and cut a leaf off and scrap out the gel inside the leaf. You may want to use a spoon to remove the gel.

Health applications

Anti-everything:

The aloe vera plant has anti-bacterial, anti-inflammatory, anti-oxidant, anti-microbial, anti-pyretic (against fevers), anti-septic, anti-fungal, and anti-viral properties. There is many properties within this plant such as sulfur, phenol, urea, nitrogen, salicyclic acid, lupeol, and cinnamic acid that will help fight off disease and protect your bodies cells.

Boosts immunity:

This plant will help to boost your body's immune system. The white blood cells are stimulated by the working components within the aloe vera to help them fight against viruses. Free radicals will be reduced due to the anti-oxidant properties.

Cardiovascular health improvements:

It has been suggested in studies that using aloe vera extracts can help to improve the speed of which oxygen is transported in your blood system. Cholesterol can also be reduced by taking in a diluted and mixed juice of the plant.

Helps to heal burns:

Adding aloe vera to the burned skin can help to speed up the healing process.

Lemon Balm

This is a herb that is named after its smell—it smells like lemons. Lemon balm is very easy to grow. It is a quick growing plant that can adapt to many types of circumstances.

To avoid unwanted spread of the plant remove the flowers. Lemon balm is used as a great flavoring in foods. It is often used in ice-creams and teas.

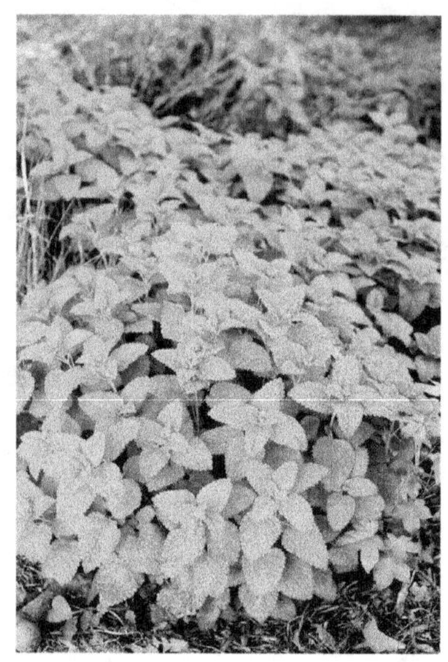

How to Grow

Lemon balm is a perennial plant which means it can grow more than one season. It grows in all kinds of soils. It prefers clay or sand-type soils. It tends to prefer a drier climate. You can put it into soil that is a little acidic between 6.0-7.5 pH level is fine.

It will grow to be about 18 inches. The best time to plant seedlings is in early spring. You might want to start growing a few seedlings in a pot indoors. Place seedlings about 15 inches apart. Plant in full sun in dry soil. Harvest time for this plant is year-round. You remove the leaves and then you can store them. Dry the leaves and store them in airtight container. You can use a distiller to remove essential oils from this plant as well as others.

Health Applications

The lemon balm herb has many health benefits from various working components within the leaves.

Calming and soothing the mind:

Often used as part of aromatherapy the scent of lemon balm is very helpful in creating a nice and calm indoor environment. Just the aroma of lemon balm essential oils will help to bring you into a calm state of mind.

Improves restful sleep:

Lemon balm can allow you to lower your overall brain activity during the peaceful state of mind you are in while sleeping. You can take lemon balm in the form of supplements.

Chapter 6. Planning an Indoor Herbal Garden

Many of us love to cook with fresh herbs because we adore the flavors they add to our culinary dishes. Below are just a few reasons why we love cooking with fresh herbs:

•   There is nothing like enjoying chopped chives over some hearty homemade soup.

•   I love throwing into my tea cup a few sprigs of fresh mint.

•   The tasty garden-fresh flavor you get when you add fresh thyme to your meals is wonderful.

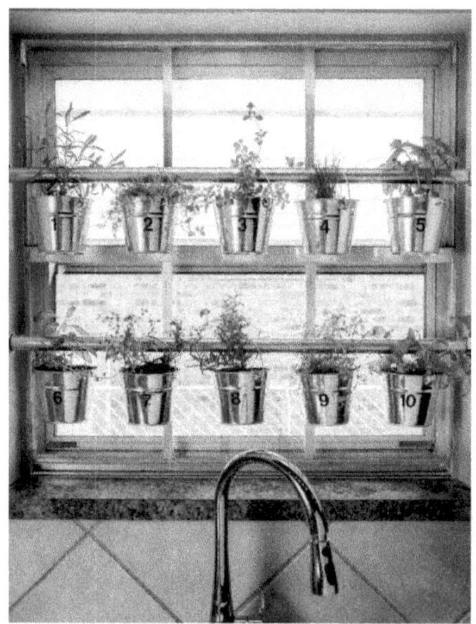

Aside from the reasons I listed above fresh herbs will enhance the flavor of many culinary dishes with their intoxicating fragrances and how they enhance the flavor of our foods. For those that do not have a garden outside, there is no need to stress you can still have your own little indoor herb garden using a few flower pots to house your herbs of choice in. You will certainly enjoy having fresh herbs all year round to add to your special dishes.

Many people that enjoy fresh herbs live in apartments or do not have access to an outside area to grow an outdoor herb garden. Using a small amount of space in your home you can grow your own fresh herbs without an outside garden. If you do not consider yourself a 'green-thumb' do not worry as many herbs basically only require a nice sunny spot in your home.

What is indoor gardening? You are going to be growing plants inside of your home. In this case it will be a selection of your favorite herbs to make yourself a small indoor herb garden. In this chapter we will take a closer look into setting up an indoor herb garden.

First pick the right location

The spot where you choose to setup your herb garden is important to the success of it thriving. Your herb garden can be grown anywhere inside your home that offers it direct sunlight.

However, the best location is the kitchen. When you are cooking up your special meals you will have easy access to your fresh herb supply. I would suggest putting it in or around your kitchen area. You want to place your herbs into containers near a window that is getting at least 5 hours of sunlight a day.

Decent Drainage

Your indoor herbs will need all the proper care that you can give them. Do not over-water your herbs. Many herbs end up dying due to their roots becoming rotted because they are soaked in water. Add your herbs to pots or containers that have good drainage to prevent root rot from occurring.

If you are growing your herb garden during the winter choose plastic or glazed containers as they do not dry out as quick as clay pots do. The house air is going to be dry due to the furnace running during the winter months.

Always Choose a High Quality Potting Mix

When you are cultivating your indoor herb garden always choose a quality potting soil. Using a good potting mix is just as important as sunlight in order for your herbs to grow healthy roots. The soil should have a nice fluffy and light texture to it.

In order for the roots of your herb plants to grow healthy they need air, as well as water. If the soil is too dense or too wet, it will only cause the plant roots to rot and die. Always use good potting soil for your herbal plants. Go to your local garden centre and they will be able to suggest to you some good quality choices of soil for your indoor herb garden.

A good way to spot a good quality soil is to check on the bag and read what the ingredients are. Good quality ingredients would include: peat moss, vermiculite, lime, perlite, a wetting agent that helps the soil to stay evenly humid, and some aged bark or any composted forest products. Make sure to avoid anything that has pesticides.

Most Common Herbs for Indoor Herb Garden:

Mint

You can get mint into two major variations, one is peppermint and one is spearmint. Peppermint is the stronger of the two and is also the one used on most therapeutic purposes such as helping to soothe and upset stomach. Spearmint is milder and can be used in culinary recipes.

Sage

Sage has a soft grayish-green color to it. It is a strong herb similar to rosemary and oregano. It is often used to spice meats and in vegetable dishes.

Parsley

There is two major variations in parsley. One is the Italian and the other is the curled leaf. The Italian variety is milder and is the one most often used in culinary dishes, adding a yummy fresh flavor to them.

Thyme

The leaves of the thyme plant have a powerful fragrance to them. Thyme is a classic addition used in French style cuisine. Compliments egg dishes very well, along with meats and veggies.

Oregano

Oregano is originally a herb from the Mediterranean. Mexican and Greeks alike love using it in their culinary dishes.

Chives

Chives are very similar to onions as they are from the same family. Chives grow in clusters like grass. They have long hollow leaves.

Garlic chives are widely used in many culinary dishes. Chives are a wonderful addition to add onto baked potatoes with sourcream or also with eggs.

Basil

Basil is part of the mint family. Sweet basil is often used in Italian cuisine. Sweet basil is the most widely used kind of basil in the world. The next popular kind of basil is Thai basil.

Rosemary

Rosemary is a very popular herb addition to many Mediterranean dishes. It is a kind of evergreen herb that is found in sunny climates.

All of the above mentioned herbs will all do well in an indoor herb garden. Not only will you enjoy the taste of your fresh herbs but you will also be able to enjoy the health benefits that come with them too!

Conclusion

I hope that you will find my book helpful to you in getting you started in growing your own indoor medicinal herb garden. You will get to enjoy these wonderful healing herbs not only in helping to improve your health and well-being but also to add yummy flavor to your culinary dishes.

There are so many different types of herbs to choose from, but to get you started I have chosen a few of the most common or popular herb plants for you to try growing in your home or in an outdoor garden—the choice will be yours! Just think of how nice it will be to try using some natural remedies using your own homegrown medicinal herbs as well as adding them into your meals to enhance their flavors!